Copyright © 2007, 2014 Stephen Whittaker, MA

All rights reserved. No part of this publication may be reproduced, stored in a retrieval system, or transmitted in any form or by any means, electronic, mechanical, photocopying, recording, or otherwise without prior written permission of the copyright owner, except for brief quotation included in a review of the book.

ISBN-13: 978-1495993596
ISBN-10: 1495993590

AversX® and STAMP® are registered trademarks. AversX® is a patented and licensed product and cannot be copied, or altered in any way.

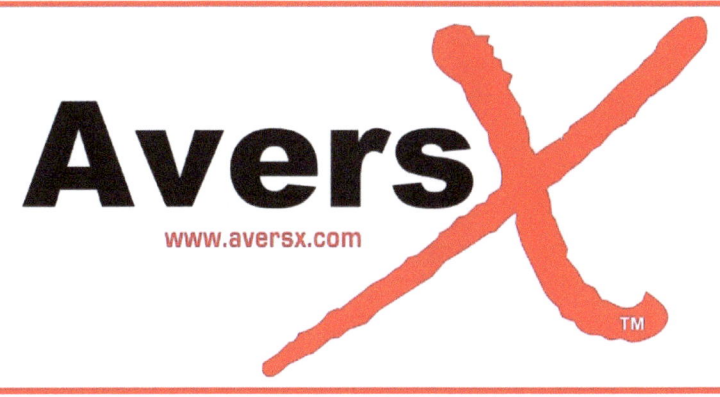

STAMP Progress Log

Name/ID:

_____

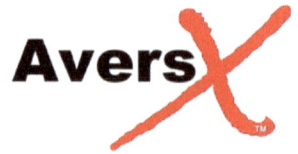 Progress Log

Day	Time	How strong of a reaction experienced	When intervention was used	What intervention was used	How Successful do you feel	What difficulties did you experience
Sunday Date:						
Monday Date:						
Tuesday Date:						
Wednesday Date:						
Thursday Date:						
Friday Date:						
Saturday Date:						

Notes:

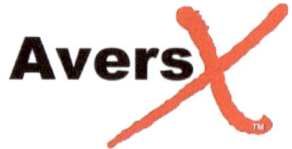 Progress Log

Day	Time	How strong of a reaction experienced	When intervention was used	What intervention was used	How Successful do you feel	What difficulties did you experience
Sunday Date:						
Monday Date:						
Tuesday Date:						
Wednesday Date:						
Thursday Date:						
Friday Date:						
Saturday Date:						

Notes:

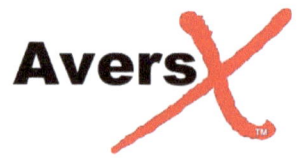 Progress Log

Day	Time	How strong of a reaction experienced	When intervention was used	What intervention was used	How Successful do you feel	What difficulties did you experience
Sunday Date:						
Monday Date:						
Tuesday Date:						
Wednesday Date:						
Thursday Date:						
Friday Date:						
Saturday Date:						

Notes:

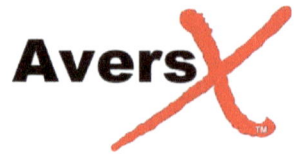 Progress Log

Day	Time	How strong of a reaction experienced	When intervention was used	What intervention was used	How Successful do you feel	What difficulties did you experience
Sunday Date:						
Monday Date:						
Tuesday Date:						
Wednesday Date:						
Thursday Date:						
Friday Date:						
Saturday Date:						

Notes:

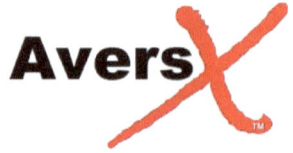 Progress Log

Day	Time	How strong of a reaction experienced	When intervention was used	What intervention was used	How Successful do you feel	What difficulties did you experience
Sunday Date:						
Monday Date:						
Tuesday Date:						
Wednesday Date:						
Thursday Date:						
Friday Date:						
Saturday Date:						

Notes:

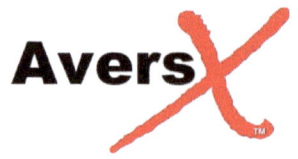 Progress Log

Day	Time	How strong of a reaction experienced	When intervention was used	What intervention was used	How Successful do you feel	What difficulties did you experience
Sunday Date:						
Monday Date:						
Tuesday Date:						
Wednesday Date:						
Thursday Date:						
Friday Date:						
Saturday Date:						

Notes:

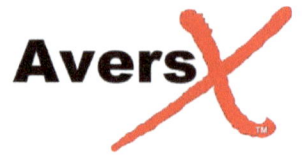 Progress Log

Day	Time	How strong of a reaction experienced	When intervention was used	What intervention was used	How Successful do you feel	What difficulties did you experience
Sunday Date:						
Monday Date:						
Tuesday Date:						
Wednesday Date:						
Thursday Date:						
Friday Date:						
Saturday Date:						

Notes:

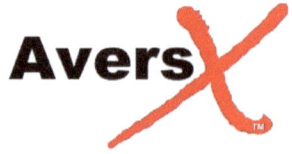 # Progress Log

Day	Time	How strong of a reaction experienced	When intervention was used	What intervention was used	How Successful do you feel	What difficulties did you experience
Sunday Date:						
Monday Date:						
Tuesday Date:						
Wednesday Date:						
Thursday Date:						
Friday Date:						
Saturday Date:						

Notes:

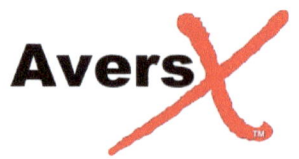 Progress Log

Day	Time	How strong of a reaction experienced	When intervention was used	What intervention was used	How Successful do you feel	What difficulties did you experience
Sunday Date:						
Monday Date:						
Tuesday Date:						
Wednesday Date:						
Thursday Date:						
Friday Date:						
Saturday Date:						

Notes:

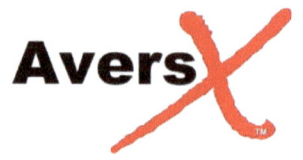 Progress Log

Day	Time	How strong of a reaction experienced	When intervention was used	What intervention was used	How Successful do you feel	What difficulties did you experience
Sunday Date:						
Monday Date:						
Tuesday Date:						
Wednesday Date:						
Thursday Date:						
Friday Date:						
Saturday Date:						

Notes:

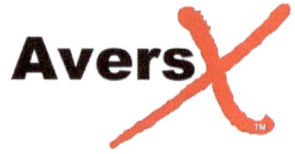 Progress Log

Day	Time	How strong of a reaction experienced	When intervention was used	What intervention was used	How Successful do you feel	What difficulties did you experience
Sunday Date:						
Monday Date:						
Tuesday Date:						
Wednesday Date:						
Thursday Date:						
Friday Date:						
Saturday Date:						

Notes:

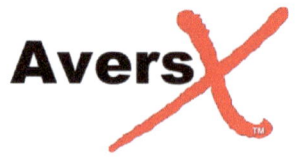 Progress Log

Day	Time	How strong of a reaction experienced	When intervention was used	What intervention was used	How Successful do you feel	What difficulties did you experience
Sunday Date:						
Monday Date:						
Tuesday Date:						
Wednesday Date:						
Thursday Date:						
Friday Date:						
Saturday Date:						

Notes:

www.ingramcontent.com/pod-product-compliance
Lightning Source LLC
Chambersburg PA
CBHW040930180526
45159CB00002BA/681